The Vegetarian Way

A Centenarian's View

Denis Malins-Smith

Harmony Kings

ISBN-13: 978-1517157852
ISBN-10: 1517157854

DEDICATION

To my son and daughter,
Roland and Suzanne.
May you enjoy reading me.

CONTENTS

*

ACKNOWLEDGMENTS

My thanks go out to Mr. Roger Byer for his keen interest and assistance.
Also, thanks to Mr. Liam and John Angus Martin for their valuable part in this venture.
And to John Miller for Internet access.

I want to acknowledge the insights from the many books, articles and other sources I have used to share my views on vegetarianism and how I've lived my life these many decades. I would especially like to acknowledge *Diet for a New America* by Mr. John Robbins; it was important to providing a world view.

*

FORWARD

This little book is not so much about health as about morality. The author passionately urges us to recognize and accept that meat-eating is wrong; that killing animals for food is wrong; that animals deserve our consideration as living beings; that the raising of animals for slaughter is damaging to our environment, and consequently also morally wrong as we are stewards of our environment. Furthermore, the social cost of eating meat is high as our global resources are squandered by making wrong communal and personal choices about what we eat.

For as long as I remember, my Dad has held to this conviction. More recent fascinating research and writing by Johnathan Safran

Foer and others, upon which he heavily relies in the following pages to justify his position, are but important endorsements of his long-held beliefs. He understands that others have made the argument thoroughly and convincingly. But the World is not listening. His fellow Grenadians are not listening. The children are not listening. And he wants to add his voice to the message, add some urgency to the message. For him, time is of the essence, as atrocities are being committed daily upon animals. And time to do so is arguably short.

You see, Dad was born in 1912, now in his 104th year, a bit late to come to the task of writing or crusading. For a man of his age, he suffers from no known ailment other than some weak knees and the need for a hearing aid. It would be natural for the rest of us to be curious as to the reasons for his longevity, and be confused by his passion for protecting animals, but we must recall that he has been the oldest living member of the RSPCA worldwide, and also a founding member of the GSPCA, a constant crusader for animal protections and rights all his life.

Without in any way attempting to distract from his singular message, I will attempt to offer some observations of his lifestyle and beliefs which may have supported his longevity, a matter of some interest to those of us who run to the doctor several times each year with one ailment or another. In the final analysis, these beliefs are commonplace and fairly fundamental. Many of us intuitively know what lifestyle changes we need to make to improve our health and longevity, but lack the discipline to do so except for the week following New Year's day. So it will come as no surprise when I say that the attribute I admire the most about him is his discipline, the virtue which makes everything else attainable, enduring and meaningful.

A search for enlightenment has been his preoccupation for as long as I can remember. Physical wellbeing, good health, appears to be a helpful condition for this spiritual journey. So diet and exercise have gone hand and hand with his search for an understanding of life. Why are we here? How can we wake up from the daily unconscious performance of routine? Can we intensify our life experience? Is there such a thing as Karma? Heaven and Hell? What is the nature of God? What role organized religion? Is our life enriched by the consideration we show for others? Need I say it, for the consideration of other living things? Vegetarianism supports both the spiritual search and the practical health imperative.

Dad is not a vegan. He eats eggs, drinks milk, enjoys cheese, but eats no meats or fish, avoids processed foods in preference to locally grown vegetables, peas and beans, corn, fruit and nuts. Such a diet is now universally recognized to reduce the probability of cancer and heart disease.

A few of his eating habits are worthy of further mention in passing. He avoids over-eating, makes a point of stopping before he is full, always recommends that one stops eating while still feeling that you can eat more. Respect your stomach, he always cautions. Chew slowly and thoroughly, enjoy your meal. He is able to eat three small meals a day and nap after the midday meal, sleep after dinner, without indigestion, GERD, or other digestive maladies. Late night snacks are not avoided, occasionally help him to sleep better. Drinking liquids with meals are minimized as he believes that this dilutes the digestive juices, impairing their work. He drinks water between meals. These steps are not by any means unusual, but helpful, and the totality of his eating habits provides a strong basis for good health.

Exercise has always been an imperative for Dad, starting from school days. Early weight training may have laid a solid foundation, followed by yoga in later years. His yoga routine is elementary yet effective, consisting of the five "Tibetan Rites" which are gaining popularity in the US and were featured on the Dr. Oz show in 2012. Another Eastern practice which has made its way to the West, the Rites are reported to enhance the seven (7) main chakras or energy centers in the body. A daily twenty-minute routine is all that he believes to be necessary; indeed he credits these exercises for making him "younger", only reducing his routine quite recently as age has taken a toll on his knees.

Dad lives for today. Long before Eckhard Tolle extolled the virtues of living in the "Now", he understood the value of presence. To explore consciousness in pursuit of that elusive enlightenment, one can only do so in the present moment. Indeed, one can only "live" in the present moment, anything else is but daydreaming about yesterday and tomorrow. And to be truly conscious of self in the moment, he has practiced meditation daily. Meditation has now become mainstream in the US and elsewhere, and is widely understood by the scientific community today to contribute to happiness, health and wellbeing. This is the "mind-body" connection referred to by Deepak Chopra, another of his favorite authors. Dad emphasizes the importance of avoiding negative thinking, as distinct from the usual recommendation of self-improvement gurus to think positively. How do you avoid negative thinking? What do you do to counter the daily concerns, worries, destructive thoughts which we all must deal with more often than not? His answer has always been to live in the moment. Once we are savoring the present, the concerns attached to memories of yesterday and the anticipation of tomorrow will fade away. This he understands to be consistent with the Christian teaching of "taking no thought for the morrow ...."

But there is much more to the health agenda. Good stewardship of the body can postpone the deterioration brought about inevitably with age, but cannot eliminate occasional discomfort. As with the rest of us, Dad is not reluctant to visit and take advice from his medical doctor when he feel it necessary, infrequent as it may be. What is interesting however is his self-healing practice of Reike. Reike is of Japanese origin, arising from the discovery that the hands can transmit life energy to parts of the body which are touched and held, need I say, in faith in the outcome, in the belief or knowledge of the healing properties of this life energy. So whenever he confronts pain or discomfort, he applies his hands to the affected area of his body and reports relief in minutes. Reike masters will tell you that each of us has the capability to do this. Dad will say that we are all part of and capable of channeling the Universal Life Force which is around and within us, and that Christ understood and used this method effectively in carrying out his healing mission on Earth.

And what is this Universal Life force if not God? Dad will tell you in amusement that God is not a man sitting on a cloud or somewhere up in space, if so they would have found Him there already. The Energy is all around us, within us, in every living thing, including of course the animals we mistakenly feed on. The Kingdom of God is within; the ground we stand on is Holy ground; He came that we may have life, and have it abundantly. Christianity, and every other significant spiritual teaching urges us to look within, to embrace life now, where in silence we may find understanding. Dad believes that Heaven may also be found within, that we may find enlightenment in this lifetime, but that very few of us do, it is in fact the ultimate challenge, the purpose of life.

Perhaps we should begin with consideration for others, for all living beings, including the animals we consume today.

Roland Malins-Smith

ONE

No man is an island unto himself. I need the tailor, the shoemaker, the mechanic, and other service providers, as they need whatever I am trained to do.

It is the same with nations, hence globalization, so that it might be safe to say that the starving millions in Africa and elsewhere, is the responsibility of the developed world, the well-off nations.

Millions of people are going without food, not because there is not enough to feed them, but because most of the grain grown goes to feed the animals–cows, pigs, lambs, chicks;

animals bred, raised and slaughtered for their flesh.

It has been reported by one observer that if 10 percent of US citizens stop eating meat, there would be no starvation on the planet.

From every conceivable angle–health, economics, environmental, starvation, animal liberation, disease prevention–there is the need to close down the slaughterhouses.

This need has been sounded loud and clear by many writers of the past, even since the beginning of the last millennium. The population of the planet appears to be growing out of control, and more and more often people are moving to the urban life, so that one writer has been calling for the provision of more slaughterhouses!

Animal flesh is the most expensive item of food, not only as it appears on the grocer's shelves, but also indirectly for the taxpayer. Governments have to subsidize the industry. It takes 16 pounds of grain to produce one pound of beef. One acre of beans or peas produces 10 to 20 times more protein than an acre of pasturage. To grow one pound of wheat requires only 60 pounds of water, whereas production of one pound of beef requires anywhere from 2,500 to 6,000 pounds of water.

An additional cost to meat eating is the degradation of the environment. "The heavily contaminated runoff and sewage from America's thousands of slaughterhouses and feedlots is a major source of pollution of the nation's rivers and streams." In 1974, the *New York Post* uncovered the shocking misuse of a valuable national resource. One large chicken slaughtering plant was found to be using 100 million gallons of water daily.

Much has been said in previous writings about the need to preserve meat with chemicals, applied also to the animals' feed, in order to fatten them and keep them alive under the harsh conditions of their confinement.

Information about modern methods of meat production refers to that obtaining in the USA where statistics are available. Unfortunately, much of the meat, including chicken, consumed in Grenada, comes from the US and New Zealand.

It is said, I think in the sacred book, "Blessed are the poor, for they shall inherit the Kingdom of Heaven." They cannot afford to eat meat!

Near to the US city of Coalingar, California, is an area several thousand acres in extent used as a collection point for thousands of cows awaiting their turn to be taken to the slaughterhouses. They are crowded in filthy conditions, so that travellers along Highway Route 5 that runs North and South of the state, have to contend with the stench in their vehicles for many a mile after leaving the vicinity.

Peter Burgwash in his book *A Vegetarian Primer*, says "I am no shrinking Violet. I played hockey and half my teeth were knocked down my throat, and I am extremely competitive on a tennis court. But that experience of the slaughterhouse overwhelmed me. When I walked out of there, I knew I would never again harm an animal. I knew all the physiological, economic, ecological arguments supporting vegetarianism, but it was firsthand experience of man's cruelty to animals that laid the real groundwork for my commitment to vegetarianism."

George Bernard Shaw wrote:

> *We pray on Sunday, that we may have light,*
> > *To guide our footsteps on the path we*
> *tread.*
> *We are sick of war, we don't want to fight.*
> > *And yet we gorge ourselves upon the*
> *dead.*

§§§§§§

"Influenced by factors ranging from health and economics to ethics and religion, millions of people around the world are turning to a vegetarian diet."

Meat eaters are trained from early age to believe that flesh foods are the most important item on the menu, and that flesh contains the type of protein that is essential to good health.

This belief is solidly engrained in most of us. As Deepak Chopra would say, it is part of the hypnosis of social conditioning, an induced fiction in which we have collectively agreed to participate.

In the process of digestion, protein breaks down into its constituent amino acids which are reconverted and used by the body for growth and tissue replacement.

"Of these twenty two amino acids, all but eight can be synthesized by the body itself and these eight amino acids exist in abundance in non-flesh foods."

"Dairy products, grains, beans and nuts are all concentrated sources of protein."

"Cheese, peanuts and lentils contain more protein per ounce than hamburger, pork or steak."

If humans were 'created' to feed on animal flesh, it would be strange that they were not also 'created' with the 'right' teeth and intestines for this purpose. Humans have teeth similar to those of herbivorous animals, teeth for biting and grinding or chewing, whereas carnivorous animals' teeth are expressly designed for tearing flesh foods.

Because of the need for flesh to pass out 'of the body' quickly before decay sets in, the carnivores have intestines only three times their length, whereas the intestines of the herbivores and those of humans have intestines 10-12 times their body length.

*

TWO

The digestive juices produced by the body of carnivorous animals are twenty times stronger than those of humans. In spite of these factors, humans insist on eating flesh foods, all the while struggling to find cures for cancer and heart disease. Some would say that meat eaters sometimes live to be centenarians. The human body, a wonderful creation, can stand much abuse. A vegetarian would not inevitably live to become a centenarian, as many other factors are involved in the process of a healthy lifestyle.

Evidence exists, however, that vegetarianism can be responsible in large measures for longevity. The Hunzas, a tribe in North India, "have become internationally known for their freedom from disease and for their long life." They are pure vegetarians. The same can be said of a village of 400 people in the mountains of Ecuador. Yet the average life span of an Esquimo is 24½ years.

As early as in 1961, the *Journal of the American Medical Association* stated that 90 to 97 percent of heart disease, the cause of more than half the deaths in the United States, could be prevented by a vegetarian diet.

Albert Einstein wrote, "It is my view that the vegetarian manner of living, by its purely physical effect on the human temperament would most beneficially influence the lot of mankind."

§§§§§§

I understand that Grenada is soon to produce chicken, meat or eggs, or both on a large scale.

If this effort is to compete with the importations from the US and Brazil, it can only do so by using their methods of mass production. This would be unfortunate, not only for the chicken, but also for the consumers, who are unaware of what goes on in a modern chicken factory, which can no longer be called a farm.

What concerns us is the cruel and unnatural way the birds are forced to live, and the extensive use of chemicals, applied to their feed in order to fatten them and to keep them alive.

As a vegetarian I am often asked, "But you eat chicken, don't you?" As though chicken is a vegetable! Actually, chickens are sentient beings, and by nature highly social animals. The author of *The Naked Ape*, Desmond Morris, has said of chickens, "Anyone who has studied the social life of birds carefully will know that theirs is a subtle and complex world, where food and water are only a small part of their behavioural needs."

In the modern chicken factory, which the directors of the huge conglomerates keep calling a 'chicken heaven', and frequently feed the schools and colleges of the US with colourful pamphlets of happy chicks, the animals live a very painful and horrible life.

At the Hainsworth 'farm' in Mt. Morris, New York, five layers (hens) are squeezed into cages 12 inches by 12 inches. The birds have great difficulty turning around. At the 345 acre 'egg city' in Moorpark, California some 2,200,000 eggs are laid daily by 3 million hens. The hens are housed five to each 16 inch by 18 inch cage.

John Robbins provides an analogy: Imagine you are in a crowded elevator with your body in contact on all sides with other bodies. Even to turn around would be difficult. This is not temporary. It is permanent, and your only release will be at the hands of the executioner. And imagine further, that the floor of the elevator is slanted sharply, so gravity tends to push you all in one direction. The floor is made of wire mesh and terribly uncomfortable to everyone's feet.

These are the conditions for the layers, which the industry tells us is "chicken heaven". Many of the chicks are unable to change position, get their claws stuck in the mesh floor, and after enough time their feet grow around the wire completing their entrapment and causing death by starvation. In order to control this, the 'farmers' cut off the toes of the young chicks!

Broilers, the name given to the chicks raised for the pot, are housed up to as many as 80,000 in one house so small that the birds get into trouble stretching their wings. The result is much fighting, causing de-feathering and death. To reduce this 'vice' on the part of the animals, the operators cut off part of their beaks, leaving a painful and inefficient eating and drinking tool for the rest of their lives. This does not end the fighting, but de-beaking as it is called in the industry, is a common practice. In further attempts to control the birds, the lighting is turned off leaving them in total darkness, and followed by light for upwards of 24 hours.

Many of the animals lose their minds and act accordingly. This is understandable when one recalls the crowing of cocks to welcome the dawn or, the chicks retiring into tree branches as the sun goes down. In the modern chicken factory they never see the light of day.

Male chicks are of little use in the provision of eggs. How they are treated after having plucked their way out of their shells, expecting to be met by the warmth of a waiting mother, is reported by an observer: "They're literally thrown away." We watched at one hatchery as 'chicken pullers' weeded out males from each tray, and dropped them into heavy-duty plastic bags. Our guide explained "we put them in a bag and let them suffocate."

Over half a million baby chicks are disposed of in this fashion every day of the year in the United States. And they are the lucky ones, because, for those chicks allowed to live, their life that follows is truly a nightmare.

And what do you think the 'lucky' chicks of 'chicken heaven' dine on? In *Scientific American*, an article reports: "The modern fowl thrives on a diet almost totally foreign to any food it ever found in nature. Its "feed is a product of the laboratory."

And a poultry man summarised the matter this way: "Virtually all chickens raised in the United States today are fed on a diet laced with antibiotics from their first day to their last. Without antibiotics, the industry could not maintain the intensive farming practices. An awful lot of them die anyway, before we can get our profit out of them. Without antibiotics, why, we'd be back to the backward practices of yesteryear."

These poor animals are riddled with disease. Due to the danger of contracting diseases from chickens, the US Bureau of Labour has listed the poultry processing industry as one of the most hazardous of occupations.

§§§§§§

The worst insults in speech are to call a man a "pig", or a woman, a "sow". This fact does not testify to the nature of pigs, but to our beliefs about them, and how far out of touch we are with these animals.

The common belief that pigs are greedy, fat, and filthy animals, without a trace of sensitivity, could hardly be further from the truth. Actually, pigs have one of the highest IQs of all animals, even surpassing the dog. They are friendly, sociable, fun-loving beings also.

W. M. Hudson, author of *Boots of a Naturalist* says of pigs: "I have a friendly feeling towards pigs generally, and consider them the most intelligent of beasts, not excepting the elephant and the anthropoid ape. I also like their attitude towards all other creatures, especially man. He is not suspicious or shrinkingly submissive like the horse, cattle and sheep, and not an impudent devil-may-care like the goat, nor hostile like the goose; nor condescending like the cat; nor a flattering parasite like the dog. He views us from a totally different standpoint as fellow citizens and brothers, and takes it for granted, or grunted, that we understand his language, and without servility or insolence, he has a natural, pleasant camarados-all or hail-fellow-well-met air with us."

We think of pigs as disgusting creatures, but Robbins believes that "what is disgusting is our attitude towards them. They are playful, sensitive, friendly animals who like to roll around and rub on things, and consider the earth their home, and not something with which to avoid contact. They wallow in mud just as stags and buffaloes do, especially in hot days when flies are troublesome. Pigs do not use mud for its own sake. They use it to cool themselves and gain relief from flies."

In recent years, pork farms are being replaced by pig factories. "Some of these are huge industrial complexes with over 100,000 pigs." There are no pig pens. "Like the chicken yard, that is a thing of the past. Every day more and more of these robust creatures are placed in stalls so cramped they can hardly move."

"If you were to look inside one of the buildings with these stalls, you would see row upon row of pigs, each standing alone in his narrow steel stall, each facing the same way like cars in a parking lot." Peter Singer and Jim Mason, authors of "Animal Factories" have described what happens to pigs' feet under these conditions: "Pigs are cloven hoofed animals, and in most, the outer half of the hoof (claw) is longer than the inner half. Outdoors the extra length is absorbed by the natural softness of the soil. On the concrete or metal floors of the factory pen, however, only the tissue in the foot can 'give'. As a result many confined pigs develop painful lesions in their feet which can open and become infected. Pigs with these foot sores usually develop abnormal postures in an attempt to relieve the pain. Eventually the crippling may worsen when the abnormal weight distribution overworks the joints and muscles in the lap, back and other parts of the pig."

One Nebraska study showed that nearly 100% of all pigs raised on concrete or metal slats had damaged feet and legs. Of course, pork producers are aware that the animals are crippled by the flooring, but they are not disturbed. So the editors of *Farmer and Stockbreeder* explained.

"The slatted floor seems to have more merit than advantage. The animal will usually be slaughtered before serious deformity sets in!" One producer summarised industry thinking: "We don't get paid for producing animals with good posture around here. We get paid by the pound."

It is difficult to imagine the suffering of today's pigs. They are crammed for a lifetime into cages in which they can hardly move, and forced against their nature to stand in their own waste. Their sensitive noses are assaulted by the stench from the excrement of thousands of other pigs. Their skeletons are deformed and their legs buckle under the unnatural weight for which they have been bred. John Robbins, author of *Diet for a New America* has noted: "I have looked into their eyes and it is a terrifying sight."

"These sensitive creatures have been literally driven mad. Forced into such bizarre conditions, the pigs are driven completely out of their minds." One reporter noted: "Some animals may become so fearful that they dare not move even to eat and drink. They become runts and die. Others remain in constant panicked motion, neurotic perversions instinct to escape. Cannibalism is common in swine operations."

According to a commentator, "A common problem in modern pork factories is 'tail biting', the action of the deranged and desperate powerful animals, driven berserk by the frustration of their natural urges. Acute tail-biting frequently results in crippling, mutilation and death. Many times the tail is bitten first, and then the attacking pig or pigs, continue to eat further into the back. If the situation is not attended to, the pig will die and be eaten."

In attempts to curb this 'vice' on the part of these animals, their tails are cut off, a practice common in the industry, and known as tail-docking. This of course is quite painful to these sentient creatures, and drives them even crazier. One pork farmer says: "They hate it. The pigs just hate it. And I suppose we could probably do without tail-docking if we give them more room, because they don't get so crazy when they have more space. With enough room they're actually quite nice animals. But we can't afford it. These buildings cost a lot."

According to John Robbins, The American Pork Queen reassures us that today's pigs receive "good feed and clean water".

He continues, "But the truth is a little different. Today, they are fed an unnatural diet to make them as fat as possible. Their feed is laced with antibiotics, sulphur drugs, and other products of the laboratory. It also features recycled waste. But if what today's pigs are fed leaves a little to be desired, it's almost a picnic compared to the water they receive to drink. Sometimes the only water they get comes from an oxidation ditch which channels wastes from factory manure pits back to the animals. They have to drink it because it's the only water offered to them."

Robbins adds that "The industry's public stance is that the health and well-being of today's pigs are better than ever, but over 80 percent of today's pigs have pneumonia at the time of slaughter. One Minnesota plant found pneumonia in the lungs of 95 percent of the pigs inspected. In 1970, 53 percent of all US pigs had stomach ulcers."

According to David Kaplan in *The Philosophy of Food*, "The Livestock Conservation Institute reports that pig producers lose more than $187 million each year from dysentery, cholera, abscesses, trichinosis, and other swine diseases. A disease known as pseudo-rabies, has been wiping out herds of factory pigs in the Midwest since 1973."

Robbins believes that "Throughout history there have been people who sensed that eating the flesh of animals, killed unnecessarily, was not the best thing we could do towards bringing peace to the world." To quote Leonardo Da Vinci, "The time will come when men, such as I, will look on the murder of animals as they now look on the murder of man."

§§§§§§

It is a common belief that most animals act instinctively, with perhaps a dash of intelligence. Robbins believes cows have a special kind of intelligence and sensitivity, and because they are such patient and gentle souls, they are thought to be dumb. They move through life with a peacefulness that is not easy to disturb.

He continues that for centuries these animals have pulled our ploughs, sweetened our soil, given milk to us. However, today these peaceful creatures have been rewarded by being treated in much the same way as today's chickens and pigs.

The US Animal Welfare Act specifically excludes creatures intended for food from its regulations governing the humane treatment of animals. "Cows, pigs and chickens are evidently not considered animals within the meaning of the act. You can be as cruel as you like, so long as the animal is going to be eaten."

"One has to wonder how the people who handle the animals rationalize what they do."

One livestock auction worker, when asked whether he was uncomfortable with the way the animals were handled, replied: "Look, if you want beef this is the way you can have it. There is no room in business for a 'be kind to animals' attitude."

Early in the last century cattle were transported by rail to the distribution depots. They came from free-range grazing, so that at least their early life was natural.

Today's cattle are shipped by trucks mostly. If you were to step inside one of these trucks you would be struck by the smell. Ventilation is almost zero. It is extremely hot in summer and severely cold in winter. The animals spend sometimes up to three days and nights without food or water.

One authority wrote: "It is difficult for us to imagine what this combination of fear, travel sickness, thirst, near starvation, exhaustion and in winter severe chill, feels like to the cattle. In the case of young calves which may have gone through the stress of weaning and castration only a few days earlier, the effect is still worse."

It is regarded by today's cattlemen as a normal part of business, that some of the animals will die in transit. It is a calculated loss. Most of the deaths are caused by a form of pneumonia known quite appropriately as 'shipping fever'. More than one animal dies of this disease for every 100 that reach market.

The Livestock Conservation Institute has called it the most costly animal disease in the United States. Livestock producers routinely use a dangerous antibiotic called chloramphenicol to treat shipping fever. It helps to keep shipping fever down and profits up.

"Shipping fever is only one cause of death of cattle in transit." Some freeze to death in winter. Others die from heat and severe dehydration in summer. Some suffocate when others pile on top of them as the over-crowded trucks go around curves.

For the animals who survive the journey, it is not 'home sweet home'. Exhausted, depleted, ill and bewildered by the harsh treatment, these peace-loving creatures may be welcomed to their new home by being dipped in a trough full of insecticides. They may be d-horned, branded, castrated, or injected with various chemicals.

And their home is now a feed lot. These feed lots are open areas fenced around to hold sometimes as many as 100,000 cows. Here, the animals are fed on a diet designed to fatten them as cheaply as possible. This may include such delicacies as sawdust laced with ammonia and feathers, shredded newspaper, edible tallow and grease, poultry litter, antibiotics, and hormones. Artificial flavours are added to trick the poor animals into eating the stuff.

Robbins adds that "The industry recognises that major health problems ensue from the way today's cattle are fed. It does not matter if the animal is ill; once it can be kept alive with drugs until slaughtered."

A cow bred for the supply of milk has no better life. Looked upon by the industry as a four legged milk pump, a machine for profit, she is bred, fed, inseminated and manipulated to a single purpose - maximum milk production at minimum cost. The average commercial cow now gives three or more times as much milk as her ancestors did. Her udder is so large, that her calves would have a hard time suckling from it if they were allowed to try. She is milked by a machine. She may spend her whole life in a concrete stall, or worst for her legs, on a slatted metal floor. She is always pregnant, and without exercise. Her nervous system becomes ragged, so she has to be given tranquillisers.

Normally she should live to be 20 or 25 years, but being so severely exploited, she would be lucky to see her fourth birthday.

*

THREE

Dairy cows are usually given hormones in order to increase their supply of milk, but under such conditions, their output drops. Then the cow, exhausted and depleted, climbs into the truck for the last journey.

In his book *Diet for a New America*, John Robbins said, "Throughout history there have been people who have chosen to be vegetarians because they did not feel it was right to kill animals for food when this was not necessary when there was other nourishing food available."

"But today, because of the way animals are raised for market, the question of whether or not to eat meat, has a whole new meaning and a whole new urgency. Never before have animals been treated like this. Never before has such deep unrelenting and systematic cruelty been mass produced. Never before has the decision of each individual been so important."

§§§§§§

There was a time when man thought the planet earth was flat and the sun moved around it. There was a time when man ate the flesh of man, and gave his brother man up for sacrifice. There was a time when folks were burnt alive for their religious beliefs.

One of these times has been referred to as the Dark Ages. I have no doubt that the present era would one day be classified as the second Dark Age, because of the systematic and unrelenting cruelty to animals being mass-produced today.

The suffering of sentient beings today is only one aspect or result of the demand for flesh foods. The cutting down and destruction of the rain forest, the disappearance of the valuable top soil, the poisoning of streams, rivers and seas, the starving millions of people, the suffering of so many from avoidable diseases, and the extinction of thousands of animal species, are all resulting directly and indirectly from the demand for flesh foods and animal products.

In the 1970s, a number of studies were published in the *Journal of the National Cancer Institute* which reported what was then startling news. Researchers were finding that the incidence of colon cancer was high in precisely those regions where meat consumption was high, and low where meat consumption was low. It was found in fact, that there is not a single population in the world with a high meat intake which does not have a high rate of colon cancer. Even the conservative journal of *The American Association for the Advancement of Science* concluded: "Populations on a high meat, high fat diet are more likely to develop colon cancer than individuals on vegetarian or similar low meat diets.

The Executive Director of the Centre for Science in the Public Interest, Michael Jacobs, has said: "Dietary fat and cholesterol speed the development of some of the most dreaded diseases, and contribute to hundreds of thousands of deaths a year.

"These diseases include coronary heart disease, peripheral atherosclerosis, gangrene, hearing loss, cancer of the breast and colon, and cerebral haemorrhage. Over the years the 'Fat Lobby' (the meat and dairy and egg industries and political allies) has not only influenced the US nation's food and nutritional policies, it has determined those policies."

According to John Robbins, meat, dairy products and eggs, are the chief source of dietary saturated fat. Along with fish, they are the only source of dietary cholesterol.

The American Journal of Clinical Nutrition reported a study in which 20 diabetics, all of whom needed insulin, were put on a high fibre very low fat diet. After only 16 days, 45 percent of these patients were able to discontinue the insulin injections.

According to Robbins, "Other studies have produced similar results. Approximately 75 percent of diabetics, who have needed insulin therapy and pills, can be freed from their need for medication in a matter of weeks on a low fat high fibre diet."

"Evidence that atherosclerosis was not a consequence of growing old, but was rooted in our dietary intake of saturated fat and cholesterol, came from the Korean War. After soldiers killed were autopsied, medical researchers were stunned by what they found. More than 77 percent of the American soldiers had blood vessels already narrowed by atherosclerosis deposits, while the arteries of the equally young soldiers of the opposing forces showed no similar damage. After putting a larger group of Korean soldiers on a US Army diet, they rapidly developed significant increases in their blood cholesterol levels."

In 1970, Dr. Ancel Keys of the University Of Minnesota School of Public Health published the results of a study involving 20,000 men in Finland, Greece, Italy, Japan, the Netherlands, the United States and Yugoslavia. Of these nations, the United States had the highest consumption of animal products, the highest consumption of cholesterol - and the highest death rate from heart disease.

One study at Loma Linda University in California involving 24,000 people, found that heart disease mortality rates for lacto-ovo-vegetarians was one third of that of meat-eaters. Another study at California Loma Linda University involving over 6,500 men, found that those who consumed large amounts of meat, cheese, eggs and milk, had 3.6 times the incidence of prostate cancer as men who ate those foods sparingly or not at all.

John Robbins in his *Diet for a New America*, has noted: "As startling as this increase in saturated fat is, it is actually small potatoes compared to far more ominous changes that have occurred in today's meats, dairy products, and eggs."

"Today's factory farm livestock are subjected to vast quantities of toxic chemicals and artificial hormones. Residues are then transmitted to the people who eat their flesh and drink their milk."

"Hardly any of these chemicals existed before World War II, as we are still to witness the long-term consequences of eating the products of factory farms which invariably contain residues from pesticides, hormones, growth stimulants, insecticides, tranquillisers, radioactive isotopes, herbicides, antibiotics, appetite stimulants, and larvicides."

*

FOUR

When the Indian people were forced to sell their land by the white man, the great chief Seattle did not ask for anything for his people or for himself. His one request was prophetic: "I will make one condition, the white man must treat the beasts of the lands as his brothers, for whatever happens to the beast soon happens to man. All things are connected."

§§§§§§

In the Western world, there is a strong belief, that "enough" protein from animal flesh, eggs and other dairy products is essential to sound healthy nutrition.

However there is "enough" scientific evidence extant today, proving this to be a fallacy. Nothing could be further from the truth. Yet most of us are quite firmly entrenched in the idea of the importance of animal protein.

It is interesting to note that this belief in the value of animal protein arose from the experiment with rats. In 1914, according to Robbins, "when Osborne and Mendel did some of the earliest laboratory researches on protein requirements," they "found the rats grew faster on animal protein than they did on protein from plants." Following this, "investigators begin to classify protein in meat, eggs, and dairy foods as "Class A" protein and plant origin protein as "Class B.""

There was no say to duplicate the above experiment on human subjects. So while the optimum amino acid pattern for rat growth was known, there was no equivalent information for human beings.

Nevertheless the Egg Board, The Dairy Council, The Livestock And Meat Board and other organisations whose purpose was to promote the sale of animal products, seized the opportunity to declare the value of their products protein-wise. Through their well-funded efforts, the idea that animal protein was superior to vegetable protein became virtually the official Nutrition Doctrine of the United States.

An editorial in the medical journal *The Lancet* has reported: "Formerly vegetable proteins were classified as second-class and regarded as inferior to first-class proteins of animal origin, but this distortion has now been generally discarded."

The Food and Nutrition Board of the National Academy of Sciences spoke of people who consume no dairy products, meats, or eggs: "Pure vegetarians from many populations of the world have maintained excellent health."

Albert Einstein said: "Nothing will benefit human health and increase chances of survival of life on earth as much as the Evolution to a vegetarian diet."

ABOUT THE AUTHOR

In 1928 at the age of sixteen years I left the Grenada Boys Secondary School without a certificate. But studying with the help of books and friends I managed to get a Cambridge Junior Certificate.

On leaving school I took a job selling hardware in St. George's, and after the boss passed away, I found myself head of the department.

After a few years of that, I joined the Public Works Department as the foreman of works. This involved repairs to all government buildings in Grenada. Not knowing much of construction, I read a lot, took a correspondence course, and learned much from the carpenters, masons, and

49

others I employed. In those days there was no qualified civil engineer in Grenada. Still, I was involved in the construction of school buildings, bridges, offices, and sea defences.

On the soft side, I played football, lifted weights, and rode on the cycle velodrome. I also did bee-keeping for a few years.

But nothing could compare to my love of music. As a trumpeter I have played with the Police Band, and the Harmony Kings, my brother Bert's band.

As the only one among the Harmony Kings still alive, I reminisce about the only recording of the band that was made, the 2007 commemorative release of "Dance Music of the Past: The Harmony Kings Orchestra".

We took our band to Trinidad in 1938 to compete with a band from Guyana, which never showed up. So we went to Sa Games Studio where Decker Records of New York was recording local music. When the calypso singers heard the Grenada band, they asked us to record their songs with our music, and we agreed.

We played for two dances and a birthday party before returning to Grenada. Then, because of World War II, members of the band went away and the Harmony Kings was no more.

After 68 years, Dr. Donald Hill of the USA sent me a copy of the CD with our music. It is now spread all over the world.

Our six recordings, as well as accompanying calypsonians Lord Executor, The Roaring Lion and The Caresser became part of the now famous "West Indian Rhythm: Trinidad Calypsos on world and local events featuring the censored recordings, 1938-1940."

I became a vegetarian after reading about its advantages. As to my longevity, 103 years at present, that is in the hands of the gods.